Ready Notes

to accompany

Comprehensive School Health Education

Totally Awesome Strategies for Teaching Health

Third Edition

Linda Meeks
Ohio State University

Philip Heit
Ohio State University

Randy Page
University of Idaho

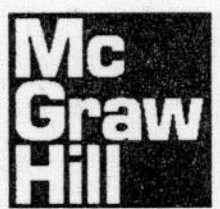

Boston Burr Ridge, IL Dubuque, IA Madison, WI New York San Francisco St. Louis
Bangkok Bogotá Caracas Kuala Lumpur Lisbon London Madrid Mexico City
Milan Montreal New Delhi Santiago Seoul Singapore Sydney Taipei Toronto

The McGraw·Hill Companies

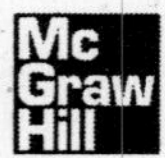

Ready Notes to accompany
COMPREHENSIVE SCHOOL HEALTH EDUCATION
Linda Meeks, Philip Heit, Randy Page

Published by McGraw-Hill, an imprint of The McGraw-Hill Companies, Inc., 1221 Avenue of the Americas, New York, NY 10020.

2 3 4 5 6 7 8 9 0 QPD/QPD 0 9 8 7 6 5 4 3 2

ISBN 0-07-283030-1

www.mhhe.com

Chapter 1

A Nation at Risk:

The Need for Comprehensive School Health Education

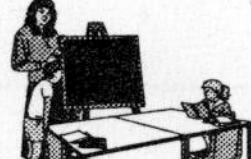

6 Categories of Risk Behavior for Today's Students

Identified by the Center for Disease Control & Prevention

- Behaviors contributing to unintentional/ intentional injuries
- Tobacco use
- Alcohol and drug use

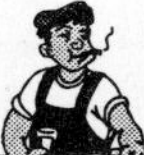

Risk behavior = action a person chooses that threatens health

6 Categories of Risk Behavior for Today's Students (cont'd)

Identified by the Center for Disease Control & Prevention

- Sexual behaviors resulting in unintended pregnancy and STD's
- Dietary patterns leading into disease
- Lack of physical activity

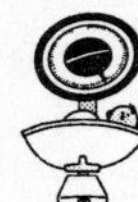

Risk behavior = action a person chooses that threatens health

Unintentional Injuries

Leading cause of death for teens

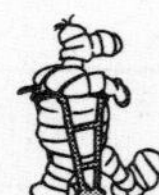

- Motor vehicle related injuries
- Fires
- Drowning
- Falls, suffocation, poisoning, etc.

Intentional Injuries

Involving interpersonal violence and self-directed violence

- Domestic violence (i.e., child abuse)
- Bullying and fighting
- Homicide
- Suicide

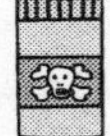

Tobacco Use

- Cigarettes, pipes, cigars, or smokeless tobacco
- Most preventable cause of death in the U.S.
- 38.6% male and 32.7% female are smokers (1999 Youth Risk Behavior Survey)
- 70% of adolescents who smoke regret having started (Office on Smoking & Health 1998)
- Depression linked to smoking (Anda et al, 1999)

Alcohol/Drug Use

- Average age of students who start to drink is between 12-13
- Drug use has increased in grades 8, 10, 12
- 47.2% of high school students have tried marijuana (Kahn et al., 2000)
- Gateway drug to other illicit drugs

Sexual behaviors Contributing to Unintended Pregnancy & STD's

- 49.9% of high schoolers report sexual intercourse experience
- Early sexual experience increases risk of pregnancy and STD's
- HIV infection of 12-21 year olds are increasing

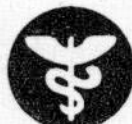

Sexual behaviors Contributing to Unintended Pregnancy & STD's (cont'd)

- Teens are at higher risk for STD's due to the likelihood of multiple sex partners
- U.S. has one of the highest adolescent birth rates among developed nations

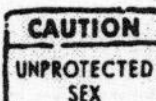

Dietary Patterns that Contribute to Disease

- Chronic diseases are linked to poor eating habits
- More young people do not meet recommendations for healthy eating
- Excess calories lead to obesity which has doubled for adolescents (Mokdad et al., 1999)
- Adolescents and children often skip breakfast which affect performance

Insufficient Physical Activity

- Physical activity is body movement from skeletal muscles which lead to energy expenditure
  - *Many young people do not get enough physical activity*
  - *Fewer children are enrolling in daily P.E.*
  - *Use of TV and video games contribute to this pattern*

Healthy People 2010 (Table 1-1)

- Represents ideas of organizations and individuals concerning the nation's health
- Two goals set by Healthy People 2010
  - *increase quality and years of healthy life*
  - *eliminate health disparities*

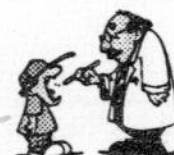

CDC School Health Guidelines

- Intended to help personnel working in schools and community-based programs meet national health objectives
  - Guidelines to:
    - *prevent the spread of AIDS*
    - *prevent tobacco use and addiction*
    - *promote lifelong healthy eating*
    - *promote physical activity among young people*

The Coordinated School Health Program

1. Comprehensive school health education
2. School health services
3. Healthful and safe school environment
4. Physical education

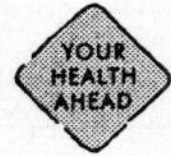

The Coordinated School Health Program (cont'd)

5. Nutrition services
6. Counseling, psychological, social services
7. Health promotion for staff
8. Family and community involvement

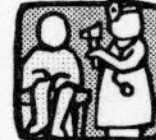

The Meeks Heit Umbrella of Comprehensive School Health Education (Figure 1-2)

Designed to protect youth from the risk behaviors by using 10 areas which young people need to improve

1. Mental/emotional health
2. Family/social health
3. Growth and development
4. Nutrition
5. Personal health/physical activity

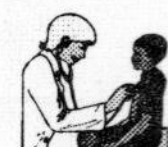

The Meeks Heit Umbrella of Comprehensive School Health Education (Figure 1-2) (cont'd)

Designed to protect youth from the risk behaviors by using 10 areas which young people need to improve

6. Alcohol, tobacco, drugs
7. Communicable and chronic diseases
8. Consumer/community health
9. Environmental health
10. Injury prevention and safety

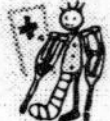

Implementing the Comprehensive School Health Education Curriculum

- Qualified and trained teachers
- Standards-based curricula and assessment
- Addressing the needs of diverse learners
- Integrating health content into other subject areas
- Using principles of effective Health Education Curricula

Chapter 1

A Nation at Risk:

The Need for Comprehensive School Health Education

Chapter 2

School Health Services:

Promoting and Protecting Student Health

School's Role in Providing School Health Services

- Promote and protect the health of students
- Services include:
  - *Health checks*
  - *Screenings*
  - *Referrals*

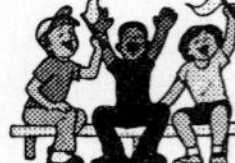

Teacher's Role with Health Services

- Observation of students
- Detect students' needs
- Offer supporting role even in emergencies
- Intervene when necessary

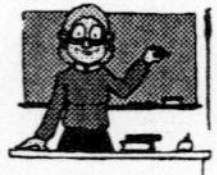

School Nurse Role with Health Services

- Advocate for staff and students
- Protect
- Promote
- Educate

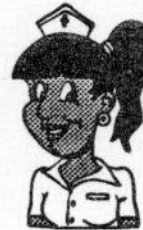

Ideally, a school nurse should be in every school

Confidentiality of Student Health Information

- Family education rights and privacy act
  - *Establishes confidentiality of all students' information, records, and rights of parents to access this*
  - *Families do not have to disclose certain health conditions to school staff (i.e., HIV status)*

Community Partnerships

- Can increase capacity to offer more services
- Families, community organizations, businesses, etc.
- Full service schools involve community partnerships between school and community agencies (21st Century Learning Centers)

School Based Health Centers

- Provide on-site comprehensive health care for young students
- Exist in 2% of all U.S. schools
- Provision of reproductive health can be opposing
- Oregon is the only state with more school-based clinics
- Such centers can reduce overall costs with healthcare

Accommodations for Special Students

- Rights of students with disabilities are protected (Rehabilitation Act of 1973)
- Schools must make provisions to accommodate students
- Teachers may be responsible for administering these services (i.e., administering medications)

Emergency Care in Schools

- Procedure plans must be in place (hierarchy of staff)
- Training must be provided (certifications)
- High-risk students are identifiable

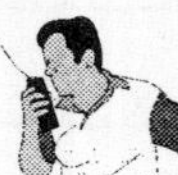

Emergency Care in Schools (cont'd)

- First aid kit is current and accessible
- Understand limitations and scope of one's abilities (i.e., DNR and information provided, first aid manual)

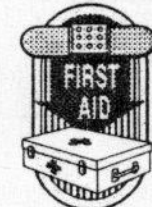

Chapter 2

School Health Services:

Promoting and Protecting Student Health

Chapter 3

A Healthful and Safe School Environment:

Protecting the Health and Safety of Students, Faculty, and Staff

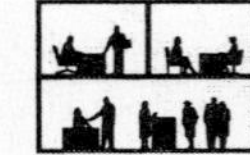

School Environments

- Multitude of dynamic conditions that are external to the person
- Two types
  - *Supportive: creates healthful choices or protects the well being of the student*
  - *Non-supportive: detracts from commitment for healthful behavior*

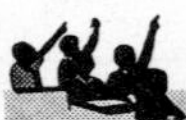

7 Physical Conditions Necessary for Optimal Learning & Development

1. School size
2. Lighting
3. Color choices
4. Temperature/ ventilation
5. Noise control
6. Sanitation/ cleanliness
7. Accessibility

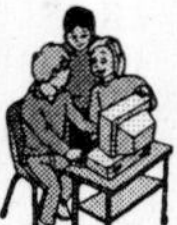

Emotional Environments

- Feelings, expectations, experiences that affect students' development
- Warm and non-threatening learning environments promote health and learning
- Teacher's personality and behavior determine emotional climate

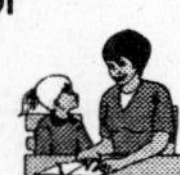

Emotional Environments (cont'd)

- Affirmative behaviors build emotional security
- Sensitivity to differences and effective classroom management can promote student achievement and self-control

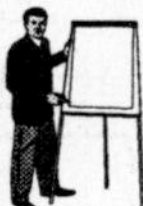

Responsibility for Health is Shared by All

- Teachers
- Students
- Parents
- Community
- Government

Teacher's Responsibilities

- Proper reporting of accidents/injuries
- Assessing/correcting potential safety hazards
- Providing proper first aid when needed
- Establishing safety procedures in the classroom
- Providing appropriate supervision of students at all times

Prevent negligence: failure to act reasonably prudent

Protecting Students' Health and Safety

- School violence
- School security measures
- Sexual harassment
- Drug use
- Tobacco use
- Bloodborne pathogens

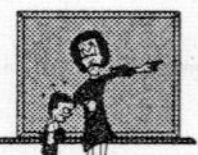

Providing Proper Nutrition

- Shared responsibility among all community members
- School food service should serve healthful foods
- Following guidelines, such as the food pyramid, provide low-cost funding for students

Health Promotion for Staff

- Rationale: higher health costs response to
  - *Decreased health care costs for staff*
  - *Decreased absenteeism*
  - *Increased job satisfaction*

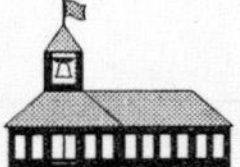

Planning and Implementing Health Promotion Programs

- Identify needs
- Use 4 components
  - *screening*
  - *education*
  - *policy/environmental changes*
  - *EAP*
- Maximize participants

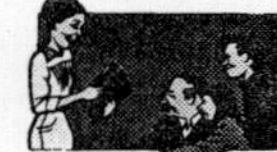

Chapter 3

A Healthful and Safe School Environment:

Protecting the Health and Safety of Students, Faculty and Staff

Chapter 4

The Comprehensive School Health Education:

A Blueprint for Implementing the National Health Education Standards

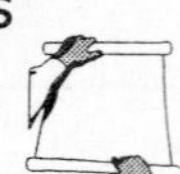

Framework for the Curriculum

National Health Education Standards

- Ensure commonality of purpose/consistency
- Improve student learning
- Provide foundation for student assessment
- Provide foundation for curriculum development
- Provide enhanced teaching preparation and continuing education

Health Literacy

- Competence in:
  - *Critical thinking and problem solving*
  - *Self-directed learning*
  - *Responsible and productive citizenship*
  - *Effective communication*

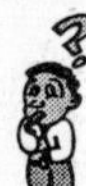

The National Health Education Standards

Standards that specify what students should know and be able to do, such as knowledge and skill develop ment

(Joint Committee on Health Education Standards, 1995)

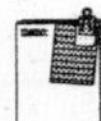

7 Health Education Standards

Students will . . .

1. Comprehend health promotion and disease prevention concept
2. Demonstrate ability to access health information and services
3. Practice health behaviors to decrease risks
4. Analyze the influence of culture, media, and other health factors

7 Health Education Standards (cont'd)

Students will . . .

5. Demonstrate interpersonal skills and communication to enhance health
6. Demonstrate the ability to goal set and make proper decisions
7. Demonstrate the ability to become a health advocate for others

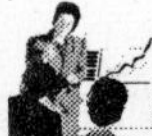

Domains of Health

- Definition of health – quality of life including the following domains:
  - *Physical*
  - *Mental/emotional*
  - *Family-social*
- Definition of wellness – another description of quality of life which encompasses the above domains of health (figure 4-1 refers to the Wellness Scale)

Model of Health and Well-Being

Includes the 3 domains of health and 10 content areas

- Mental/emotional health
- Family/social health
- Growth/development
- Nutrition
- Personal health/activity
- Alcohol, tobacco, drugs
- Communicable and chronic diseases
- Consumer/community health
- Environmental health
- Injury prevention and safety

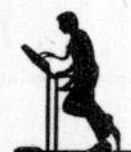

Performance Indicators

1. Understanding the relationship to behavioral objectives
2. Developing behavioral objectives
3. Classifying behavioral objectives

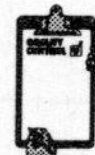

How to Teach Health Education Standards 1-7

1. Comprehend health facts
2. Access valid health information, products, and services
3. Make health behavior contracts
4. Analyze influences on health

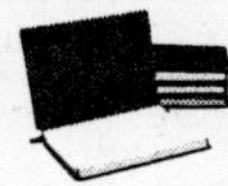

How to Teach Health Education Standards 1-7 (cont'd)

5. Communicate in healthful ways
6. Set health goals and use responsible decision-making model
7. Be a health advocate

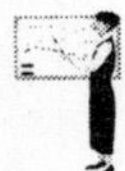

Assessment Techniques

- Opportunity to learn standards
- Curriculum
- Students

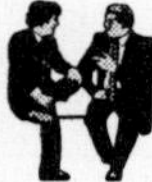

Chapter 4

The Comprehensive School Health Education:

A Blueprint for Implementing the National Health Education Standards

Chapter 5

Instructional Strategies and Technologies:
Motivating Students to Learn

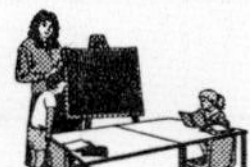

Instructional Strategies

1. Lecture
2. Lecture and discussion
3. Role play
4. Brainstorm
5. Buzz groups

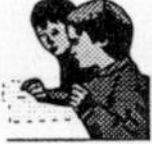

Instructional Strategies (cont'd)

6. Panel discussions
7. Debate
8. Cooperative learning
9. Decision making
10. Self-appraisals and health behavior inventories

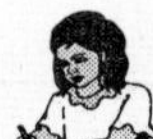

Instructional Strategies (cont'd)

11. Student presentations
12. Field trips
13. Demonstrations
14. Guest speakers

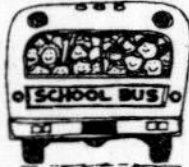

Educational Technologies

- Hardware
- Software
- Telecommunications
  - *Email*
  - *www*
  - *Chat*
  - *Bulletin boards*
  - *Discussion groups*

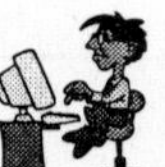

Educational Technologies (cont'd)

- Multi-media
- Virtual reality

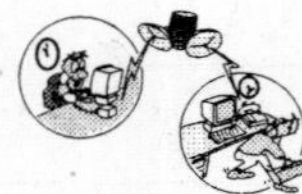

Chapter 5

Instructional Strategies and Technologies:

Motivating Students to Learn

Chapter 6

Mental and Emotional Health

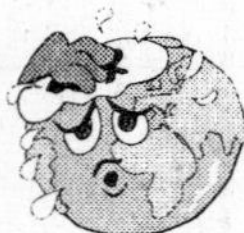

Wellness – 10 Factors

Quality of life that results from your health status

1. Heredity
2. Quality of environment
3. Random life events
4. Your health care
5. Chosen behaviors
6. Quality of relationships
7. Decisions made
8. Use of resistance skills
9. Risks taken
10. Resiliency factors

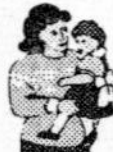

Life Skills

- Self-responsibility/discipline
- Health behavior inventories
- Health behavior contracts
- Rewards

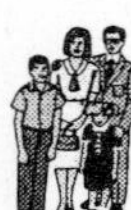

Health Knowledge – 10 Areas

Information gained on health

1. Mental/emotional
2. Family/social
3. Growth/development
4. Nutrition
5. Personal health/activity
6. Alcohol, tobacco, drugs
7. Communicable diseases
8. Consumer/community health
9. Environmental
10. Injury prevention/safety

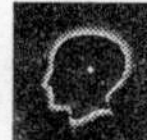

Decision-Making Styles

- Inactive (procrastinate)
- Reactive (others decide)
- Proactive (empowered by self)

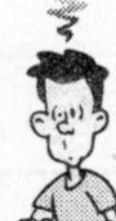

Resistance Skills

Skills that allow the "no" concept

- Factors affective resistance
  - Self-confidence
    - *belief in oneself vs. aggressive or passive behaviors*
  - Assertive behavior
    - *honesty without threat*

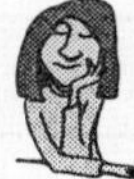

Good Character Skills

- Obtaining values (standard)
- Character (self-control)
- Moderation (limits)
- Delayed gratification (voluntary)
- Positive self-esteem (self-worth)

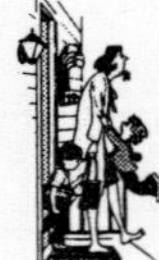

Promoting Mental Alertness/ Health Mind

Avoid addictions (engaged in compelling behavior)

Drug	Tobacco	TV
Eating	Perfectionism	Thrill seeking
Exercise	Relationship	Work
Gambling	Sex	Shopping

Mental Disorders

- Affective
- Anxiety
- Dissociative
- Personality
- Somatoform
- Schizophrenia

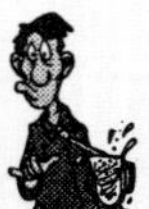

Expressing Emotions

- Communication (I, You)
- Active listening
- Non-verbal
- Understanding anger control and management

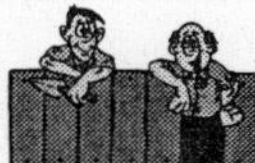

Understanding Stress

- Stress
- Stressor
- Eustress
- Distress

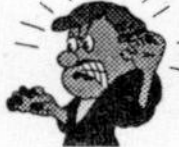

G.A.S. (General Adaptation Syndrome)

- 3 steps
  - Alarm
  - Resistance
  - Exhaustion

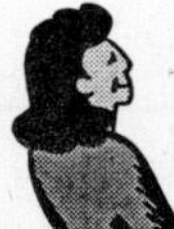

Resiliency Skills

- Deny
- Anger
- Bargain
- Depression
- Acceptance

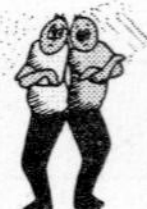

Anger and Depression

- Can lead to:
  - *Inability to cope*
  - *Illness*
  - *Family patterns*
  - *Alcohol/drug use*
  - *Suicide attempts (parasuicide)*

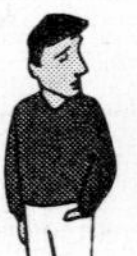

Chapter 6

Mental and Emotional Health

Chapter 7

Family/Social Health

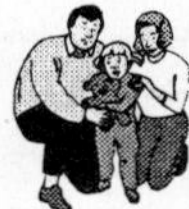

Healthful Family Relationships

- Self-respective behavior
- Healthful sexual attitudes
- Effective communication
- Clear sense of values
- Expressing love/affection
- Respect autonomy

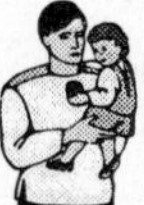

Healthful Family Relationships (cont'd)

- Responsible decision-making
- Resolving conflicts
- Effective coping skills
- Delaying gratification
- Give/receive kindness
- Work ethic

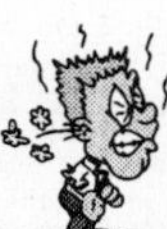

Dysfunctional Family Relationships are Destructive

- Chemical dependence
- Other addictions
- Perfectionism
- Violence
- Abuse
- Abandonment
- Mental disorders

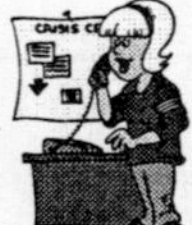

Types of Conflict

- Intrapersonal
- Interpersonal
- Intragroup
- Intergroup

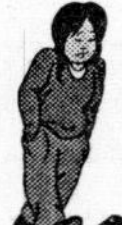

Types of Conflict Response Styles

1. Avoidance
2. Confrontation
3. Resolution/mediation

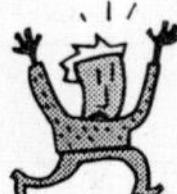

Initiating Friendship Concept

- Carry on a conversation
- Handle rejection
- Recognize shyness/loneliness
- Understand when to end a friendship

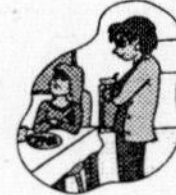

Reducing the Risk of Date Rape

- Date/Acquaintance Rape
  - Unwanted sexual advances known to t he victim
- Factors
  - *Alcohol/drugs*
  - *Communication (lack of)*
  - *Include others*
  - *Avoid isolated areas*
  - *Set rules/standards up front*

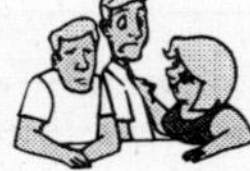

Reasons to Wait Before Having Sex

- Marriage
- STD's (i.e., HIV)
- Pregnancy
- Responsibility/character
- Respect

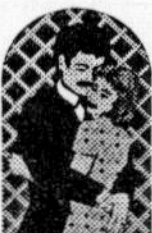

Recognizing Harmful Relationships

- People pleaser person
- Enabler
- Clinger
- Fixer
- Distancer
- Controller
- Center
- Abuser
- Liar
- Promise breaker

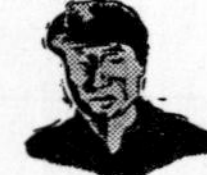

Developing Marriage Skills

- Intimacy – deep shared meaning between two people
  - Philosophical
  - Psychological
  - Creative
  - Physical

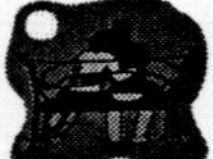

Responsible Parenting

1. Develop intimacy with child
2. Care during growth/development
3. Help with self-discipline and self-control
4. Avoid child abuse

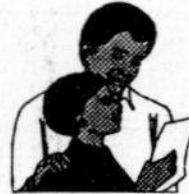

Making Healthful Adjustments to Family Changes

- Extended families
- Marital stress/conflict
- Concept of divorce
- Single custody families

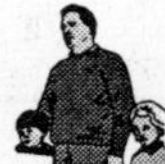

Making Healthful Adjustments to Family Changes (cont'd)

- Remarriage of a parent
- Loss of job
- Incarceration

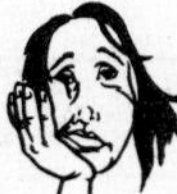

Chapter 7

Family/Social Health

Chapter 8

Growth and Development

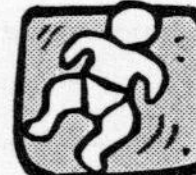

Nervous System

- Brain/spinal cord
- 2 divisions
  - CNS
  - PNS
- Parts of the brain
  - Cerebrum (largest part)
  - Cerebellum (motor activity)

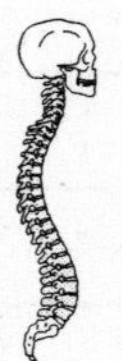

Cardiovascular System

- Components of blood (plasma, RBC's, WBC's, hemoglobin, platelets)
- Blood vessels (artery, vein, capillary)
- Heart (four-chambered pump)

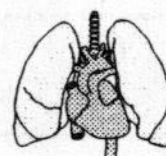

Respiratory System

- Pharynx
- Epiglottis
- Trachea
- Bronchi
- Lungs

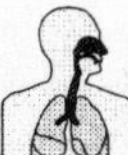

Skeletal System

- Bone (206 bones for adults)
  - Periosteum
  - Bone marrow
- Cartilage
- Ligaments

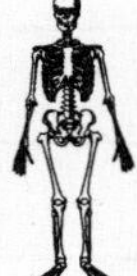

Muscular System

- Voluntary/involuntary muscle types
- 3 types
  - *Smooth*
  - *Cardiac*
  - *Skeletal*

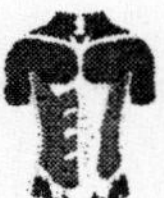

Endocrine System

- Glandular control producing hormones
  - *Pituitary*
  - *Thyroid*
  - *Parathyroid*
  - *Pancreas*
  - *Adrenals*
  - *Ovaries*
  - *Testes*

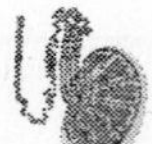

Digestive System Components

- Mouth
- Esophagus
- Stomach
- Small intestine
- Liver
- Pancreas
- Large intestine

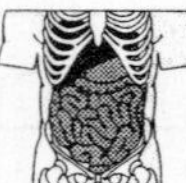

Urinary System

- Kidneys
- Ureters
- Bladder
- Urethra

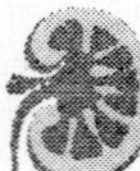

Integumentary System

- Skin
- Glands
- Hair
- Nails

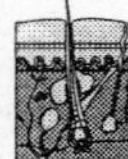

Puberty in Females

- Estrogen stimulates secondary sex characteristics
- Emotion changes
- Physical changes
- Sexual behaviors
- Menstrual cycle

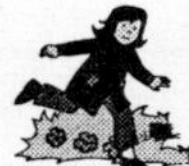

Female Reproductive System

- Ovaries
- Fallopian tubes
- Vagina (labias)
- Hymen
- Clitoris
- Cervix

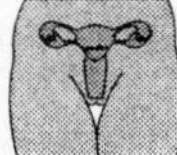

Puberty in Males

- Testosterone stimulates secondary sex characteristics
- Emotion changes
- Physical changes

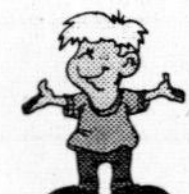

Male Reproductive System

- Penis
- Testes
- Epididymus
- Cowper's gland
- Prostate gland
- Sperm

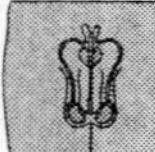

Pregnancy and Childbirth

- Understand concepts of conception and fertilization
- Identify pregnancy determination
- Understand prenatal care examples
- Know 3 stages of labor
  - *dilation of cervix*
  - *fetal expulsion*
  - *afterbirth*

Risks of Teen Pregnancy/Parenthood

- Low birth weight
- Anemia
- Toxemia

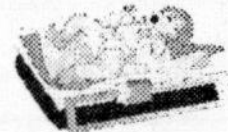

Developmental Tasks of Adolescence

- Establish friends
- Be comfortable with your gender role
- Be comfortable with your body
- Be emotionally independent from adults

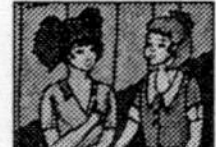

Developmental Tasks of Adolescence (cont'd)

- Learn marriage and parenting skills
- Prepare for a career
- Establish values
- Achieve social responsibility

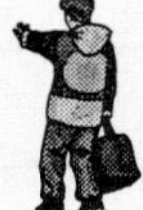

Learning Styles

- Visual
- Auditory
- Kinesthetic
- Global

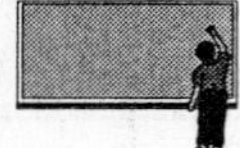

Learning Disabilities

- Dyslexia
- ADD
- ADHD
- Tracking disorder

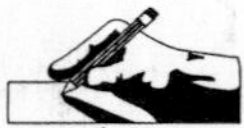

Understand Aging of the Following Systems

- Nervous
- C.V
- Immune
- Respiratory
- Skeletal
- Muscular
- Endocrine
- Digestive
- Urinary
- Integumentary
- Reproductive

Death and Dying

- Identify the following terms:
  - Life support
  - Legal death
  - Brain death
  - Living will

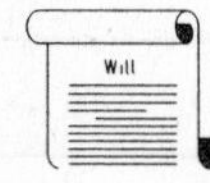

Identify 5 Stages of Grief

- Denial
- Anger
- Bargaining
- Depression
- Acceptance

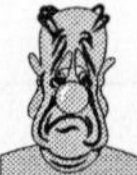

Chapter 8

Growth and Development

Chapter 9

Nutrition

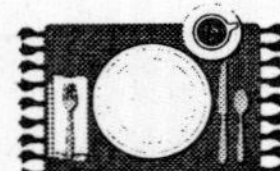

Six Nutrients

Substances that help with body processes

- Protein
- Fat
- Carbohydrates
- Water
- Vitamins
- Minerals

Calorie = unit of energy

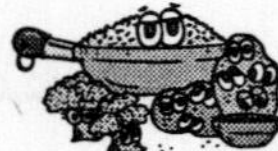

Protein

- Function – growth and repair
- Kcal value – 4 Kcal/gram
- Types – complete/incomplete
- Basic breakdown – amino acids

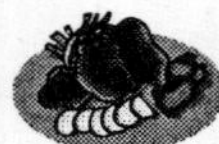

Carbohydrates

- Function – instant energy
- Kcal value – 4 Kcal/gram
- Types – single/complex
- Basic breakdown – glucose

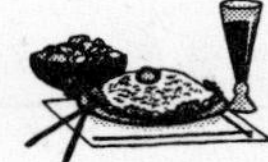

Fats

- Function – long-term energy/storage
- Kcal value – 9 Kcal/gram
- Types – saturated/unsaturated
- Basic breakdown – fatty acids

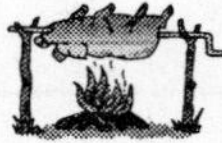

Vitamins

- Function – assists with body processes
- Kcal value – 0
- Types – water (BC) and fat soluble (ADEK)

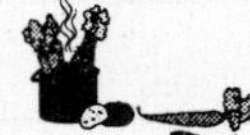

Minerals

- Function – regulates chemical reactions in body
- Kcal value – 0
- Types – macro/micro

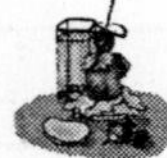

Water

- Function – waste removal, blood formation, body regulation
- Kcal value – 0
- water makes up 60% of body weight
- Recommendation 6-8 glasses per day

Food Pyramid Guide

USDA Food Guide Pyramid
Fats, Oils, and Sweets USE SPARINGLY
KEY
Fat (naturally occurring and added)
Sugars (added)
These symbols show fats, oils, and added sugars in foods.
Milk, Yogurt, and Cheese Group 2-3 SERVINGS
Meat, Poultry, Fish, Dry Beans, Eggs, and Nuts Group 2-3 SERVINGS
Vegetable Group 3-5 SERVINGS
Fruit Group 2-4 SERVINGS
Bread, Cereal, Rice, and Pasta Group 6-11 SERVINGS

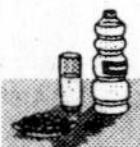

Vegetarian Diet

- Vegan
- Lacto vegetarian
- Ovo-lacto vegetarian
- Semi vegetarian

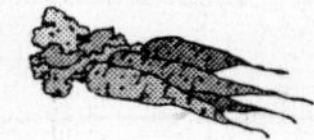

Diet and Cancer

- Avoid obesity
- Eat a variety of foods
- Include fiber

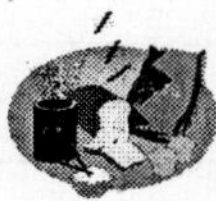

Diet and Cancer (cont'd)

- Consume foods with anti-oxidants
- Reduce fat intake
- Avoid alcohol

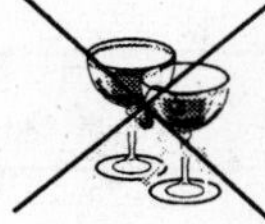

Diets and Cardiovascular Disease

- Watch for the following items:
  - Saturated fats
  - Cholesterol
  - Transfatty acids

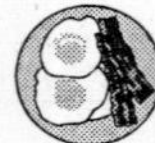

Other Disease or Conditions

- Be watchful for the following with regard to diets
  - *Diabetes*
  - *Hypoglycemia*
  - *Osteoporosis*
  - *Allergies/intolerances*

Nutrition Facts Label

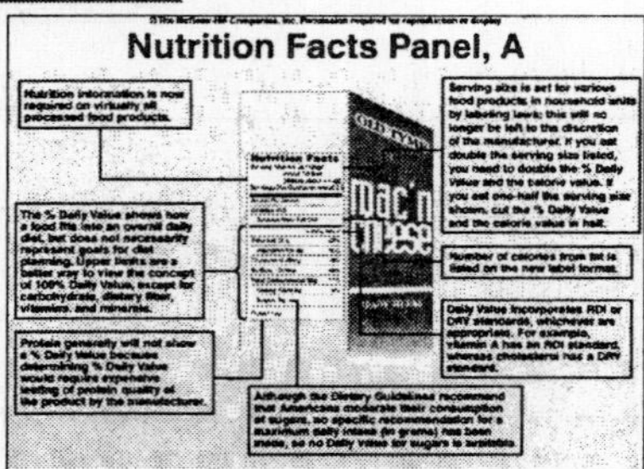

Foodborne Illnesses

- Most common to recognize:
  - *E. coli 0157:H7*
  - *Campylobacter*
  - *Salmonella*
  - *Calicivirus/Norwalk*
  - *Others: shigella, cryptosporidia, botulism*

Desirable Weight and Body Composition

- Identify these terms:
  - *Body frame*
  - *BMR (basal metabolic rate)*
  - *Desirable weight*
  - *Essential body fat*
  - *Obesity*

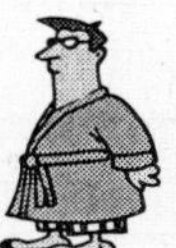

Weight Loss Strategies

- Fad diets
- Liquid diets
- Medications
- OTC products
- Diuretics and laxatives

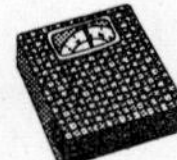

Risks for Developing an Eating Disorder

- Body image
- Sexual maturity
- Perfectionism
- Control
- Inability to express oneself

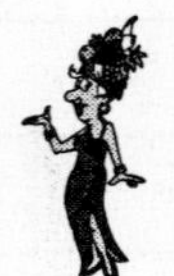

Types of Eating Disorders

- Anorexia nervosa
- Bulimia
- Binge-eating disorder

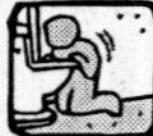

Chapter 9

Nutrition

Chapter 10

Personal Health and Physical Activity

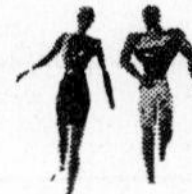

Physical Exams

- Health history
- ECG
- Urinalysis
- Blood test

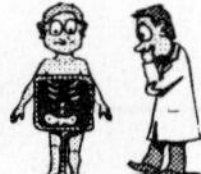

Eye Care and Conditions

- Visual acuity (sharpness)
- Refractive error (variation of eyeball):
  - *Myopia*
  - *Hyperopia*
  - *Astigmatism*
  - *Presbyopia*
- Conjunctivitis
- Glaucoma

Dental Health

- Types of teeth (incisors, cuspids, bicuspids, molars)
- 32 permanent teeth
- Check-ups
  - *Teeth cleaning*
  - *X-rays*
  - *Whitening*
  - *Sealants*
  - *veneers*

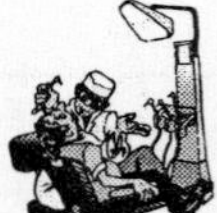

Keeping Teeth Healthy

- Brushing
- Flossing
- Fluoride
- Diet

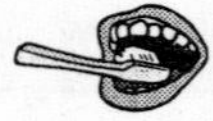

Sleep Concepts

- Types of sleep (REM, non-REM)
- Function: restoration of the mind
- Insomnia: inability to fall asleep

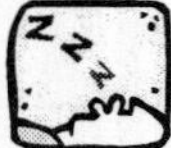

Health Benefits of Physical Activity

- Decreases risk of:
  - *Death*
  - *Cardiovascular disease*
  - *Type 2 diabetes*
  - *High blood pressure*
  - *Colon cancer*
  - *Feelings of depression and anxiety*

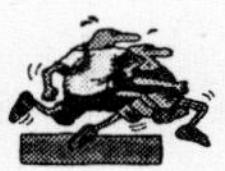

Health Benefits of Physical Activity (cont'd)

- Controls weight
- Builds/maintains bones, muscles, and joints
- Helps older adults with physical functioning
- Promotes psychological well-being

5 Health-Related Fitness Components

1. Cardiorespiratory fitness
2. Muscular strength
3. Muscular endurance
4. Flexibility
5. Body composition

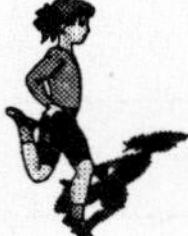

Identify the Following Exercise Terms

- Aerobic exercise
- Anaerobic exercise
- Isometric exercise
- Isotonic exercise
- Isokinetic exercise

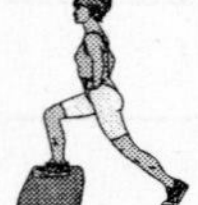

F.I.T.T.

F = *frequency* (how often)

I = *intensity* (how hard)

T = *time* (how long)

T = *type* (what kind)

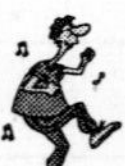

Concepts of Cardiorespiratory Fitness

- Frequency: 3-5 times/week
- Intensity: at target heart rate *(220 – age x 70-85%)*
- Time: 20-60 minutes
- Type: prolonged activity without stopping

Include warm-up and cool-down

Flexibility: range of motion around a joint

- Frequency: 2-3 times/week
- Intensity: hold for 15-30 seconds
- Time: 15-30 minutes
- Types: static and ballistic

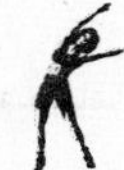

Body Composition

- Ratio of lean to fat %
- Measurement through skinfolds
- Include proper diet, physical activities

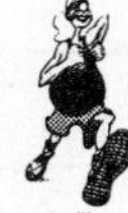

Performance-Related Fitness (Sport Skills)

- Agility
- Balance
- Coordination
- Reaction time
- Speed
- Power

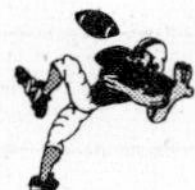

Training Principles

1. Warm-up
2. Cool-down
3. Specificity
4. Overload
5. Progression
6. Fitness reversibility

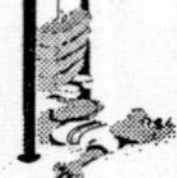

Sports Injuries Can Include . . .

- Overuse
- Microtrauma
- Bruise
- Muscle cramp
- Muscle strain

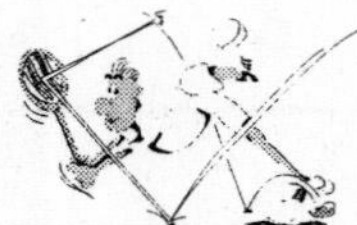

Sports Injuries Can Include . . .

- Shin splints
- Side stitch
- Sprain
- Stress fracture
- Tendonitis

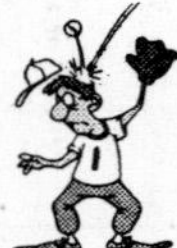

Fitness Plan

- Use F.I.T.T.
- Warm-up and cool-down
- Cardiovascular fitness
- Resistance exercises
- Flexibility exercises

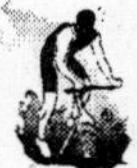

Chapter 10

Personal Health and Physical Activity

Chapter 11

Alcohol, Tobacco and Other Drugs

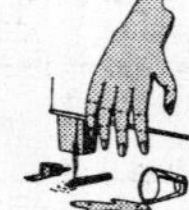

Identify the Following Terms . . .

- Drug
- Responsible drug use
- Drug misuse
- Drug abuse

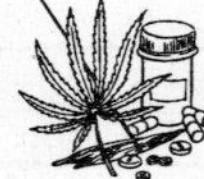

How Drugs Enter the Body

1. Mouth
2. Injection
3. Inhalation
4. Absorption
5. Implantation

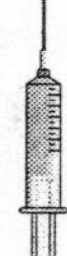

Identify the Following Concepts . . .

- Drug dependence
- Physical dependence
- Tolerance
- Withdrawal
- Psychological dependence

Co-dependence of Family Members

- Chief enabler
- Family hero
- Scapegoat
- Lost child
- Mascot

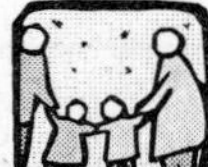

Alcohol Terms

- Fermentation
- Distillation
- Proof
- Blood alcohol concentration

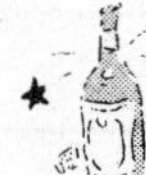

Factors Affecting BAC

1. Amount consumed
2. Rate of consumption
3. Body weight
4. Body fat %
5. Gender
6. Feelings
7. Food eaten
8. Presence of other drugs
9. Age
10. Carbonation

Effects of Alcohol on the Body

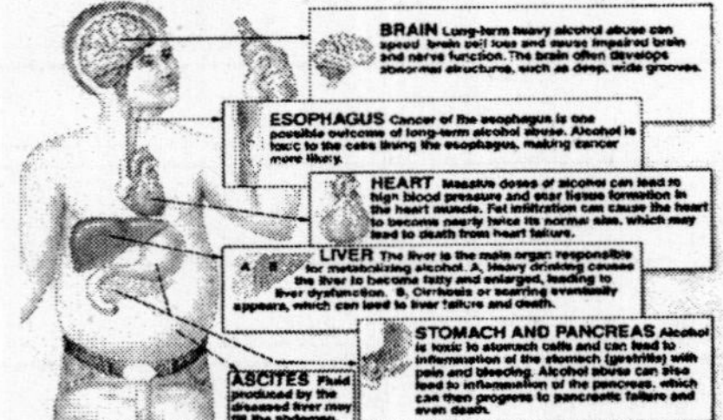

Effects of Alcohol During Pregnancy

- Miscarriage
- Stillbirth
- Low birth weight
- FAS (fetal alcohol syndrome)

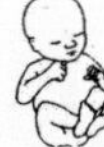

Alcohol Effects Upon Decision Making

- Wrong decisions
- False sense of confidence
- Impaired judgment
- Feelings of invincibility

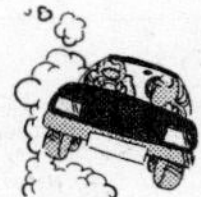

Alcohol Effects Upon Decision Making (cont'd)

- Intensified feelings
- Impaired reaction time
- Aggressive behavior
- Intensified emotions

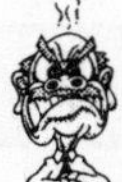

Illegal Behaviors Associated with Alcohol

- Violence
- Domestic violence
- Rape
- Suicide
- DUI
- Violation of laws

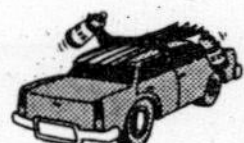

Treatment for Alcoholism

- AA (Alcoholics Anonymous)
- Al-non
- Al-teen
- Adult Children of Alcoholics (ACOA)

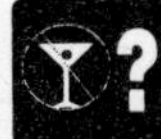

Tobacco Products Containing Nicotine

- Cigarettes
- Bidi
- Cloves
- Cigars
- Snuff

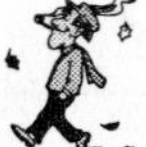

Health Consequences of Smoking

- Cancer
- Respiratory diseases
- Cardiovascular diseases
- Accidents

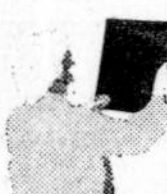

Identify Secondhand Smoke

- Environmental
- Sidestream
- Mainstream

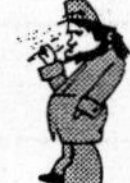

Quitting Tobacco Use

- Nicotine patch
- Nicotine gum
- Nicotine inhaler
- Nicotine spray
- Anti-depressants
- Support group/ programs

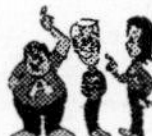

Stimulants

- Function: speeds up the CNS
- Types
  - *Cocaine*
  - *Amphetamines*
  - *Ephedrine*
  - *MDMA (ecstasy)*
  - *Caffeine*

Sedatives - Hypnotics

- Function: produces drowsiness
- Types
  - *GHB*
  - *Tranquilizers*

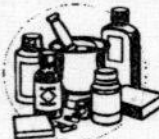

Narcotics

- Function: decrease pain
- Types
  - *Morphine*
  - *Codeine*
  - *Heroin*

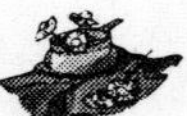

Hallucinogens/Psychedelics

- Function: interfere with senses
- Types
  - *LSD*
  - *PCP*
  - *Ketamine*

Marijuana – Cannabis Plant Containing THC

- Function: variety of psychoactive effects
- Types
  - *Hash*
  - *Hemp*

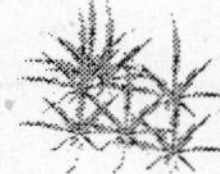

Inhalants

- Function: affects moods and behavior
- Types
  - *Household chemicals*

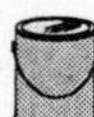

Treatment

- Detoxification
- Inpatient care
- Outpatient care
- Halfway houses
- Recovery programs

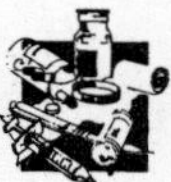

Chapter 11

Alcohol, Tobacco and Other Drugs

Chapter 12

Communicable and Chronic Diseases

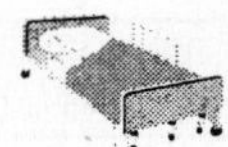

Identify 6 Pathogens

1. Bacteria
2. Fungi
3. Virus
4. Protozoa
5. Helminths
6. Rickettsia

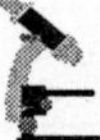

The Immune System

- Lymphocytes (B and T cells)
- Antibodies
- Macrophages
- Active/passive immunity

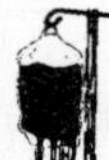

Infectious Respiratory Diseases

- Common cold
- Influenza
- Pneumonia
- Strep throat
- Tuberculosis

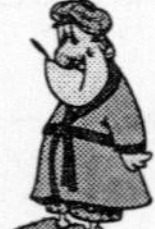

STD's

- Chlamydia
- Genital herpes
- Genital warts
- Gonorrhea
- Pubic lice
- Syphilis
- Trichomoniasis
- Viral hepatitis (A, B, C, D, E)

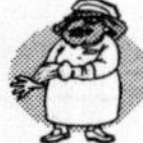

HIV Infection

- Human Immunodeficiency Virus
- Destroys T-cells
- Susceptible to opportunistic infections
- Destroys brain and nerve cells
- If <200 CD4 cells, leads to AIDS (Acquired Immunodeficiency Syndrome)

HIV Transmission

- Sexual contact with infected person
- Open mouth kissing
- Hypodermic needle contamination
- Contact with bodily fluids from infected person

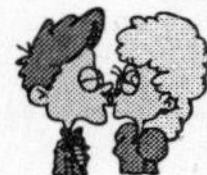

HIV Transmission (cont'd)

- Contaminated blood products
- Organ donation
- Perinatal transmission

HIV Testing

- Antibody test
  - ELISA
  - Western blot

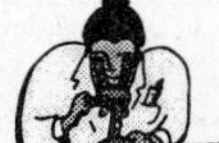

Treatment for HIV/AIDS

- Measurement of viral load determines the following:
  - *Antiretroviral drugs (i.e., HAART)*
  - *Proper diet*
  - *Rest*
  - *Exercise*

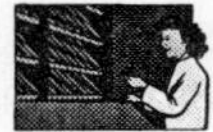

Cardiovascular Diseases

- Arteriosclerosis/ atherosclerosis
- Coronary heart disease
- Arrythmias
- Congestive heart failure
- Rheumatic fever
- Stroke

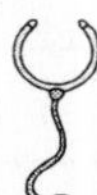

Reducing Risk of Heart Disease

- Watch cholesterol levels
- Diet containing anti-oxidants
- Avoid tobacco products
- Check blood pressure

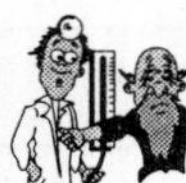

Reducing Risk of Heart Disease (cont'd)

- Exercise
- Manage stress
- Keep body fat levels healthy

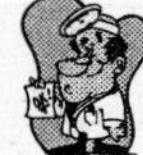

Diabetes

- Two types
  - *Type 1*
  - *Type 2*
- Gestational occurs in some females during pregnancy
- Risks include 4 F's: fat, female, family, forty

Cancer Terms

- Tumor
- Benign
- Malignant
- Metastasis

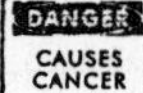

Cancer Treatment

- Radiation
- Chemotherapy
- Immunotherapy

Chronic Conditions

- Arthritis
- Cerebral palsy
- Chronic fatigue syndrome
- Cystic fibrosis
- Down syndrome
- Parkinson's disease
- Peptic ulcers
- Epilepsy
- Hemophilia

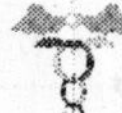

Chronic Conditions (cont'd)

- Migraine headache
- Multiple sclerosis
- Muscular dystrophy
- Narcolepsy
- Sickle cell anemia
- Lupus

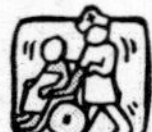

Chapter 12

Communicable and Chronic Diseases

Chapter 13

Consumer and Community Health

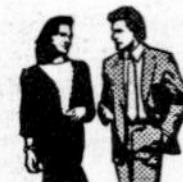

Sources of Health Information

- Mass media
- Books
- Online communication
- Healthcare professionals
- Local/state health departments
- Federal government agencies
- Community agencies

Consumer Protection

- Federal agencies
- State/local agencies
- Private organizations

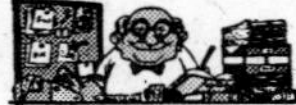

Healthcare Providers

- Physician
  - M.D.
  - D.O.
- Primary care vs. specialists

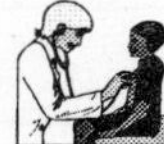

Practitioners vs. Professionals

- Healthcare practitioners
  - *Podiatrist, dentist, optometrist*
- Allied health professional
  - *Nurses, physical therapists*
  - *Under the supervision of a healthcare practitioner or M.D.*

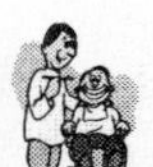

Health Careers - Professionals in the Health Field

- Physician
- Radiologic technologist
- Recreation therapist
- Registered nurse
- School psychologist
- Speech pathologist
- Audiologist
- ATC athletic trainer

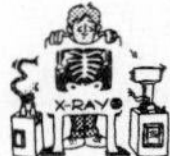

Health Careers - Professionals in the Health Field (cont'd)

- Health educator
- Dental hygienist
- Dentist (D.D.S., D.M.D)
- Dietician
- Guidance counselor
- Health education teacher
- Health services administrator

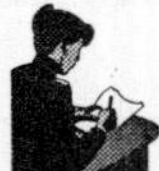

Health Careers - Professionals in the Health Field (cont'd)

- Medical writer
- Occupational therapist
- Pharmacist
- Social worker
- Pharmacologist
- Physical therapist
- Clinical psychologist
- EMT/Paramedic
- Licensed Practical Nurse (L.P.N.)

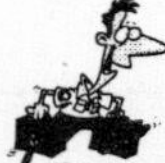

Chapter 13

Consumer and Community Health

Chapter 14

Environmental Health

Environmental Issues

- Population growth
- Poverty and hunger
- Greenhouse effect/global warming
- Destruction of ozone layer
- Destruction of rain forests

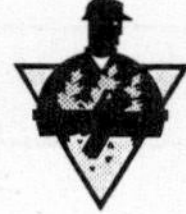

Air Pollution

- Contamination of the air
- Affects various areas of health such as respiratory, CV, immune system
- Sources
  - *Fossil fuels*
  - *Particulates*
  - *Motor vehicle emissions*
  - *Smog*
  - *Indoor air pollution*

Clean Water: Safety & Pollution

- Fresh water sources
  - Rivers
  - Streams
  - Wells
- Pollution sources
  - Toxic chemicals
  - Fertilizers
  - Trihalomethanes
  - Sediments

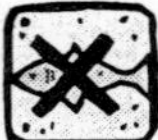

Clean Water: Safety & Pollution (cont'd)

- Pollution sources
  - Toxic chemicals
  - Fertilizers
  - Trihalomethanes
  - Sediments
  - Radioactive waste
  - Thermal pollution
  - Microorganisms

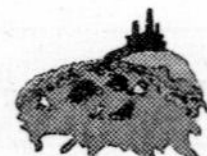

Waste Disposal Terms

- Solid waste
- Landfill
- Precycling
- Recycling
- Incineration
- Composting
- Deep-injection wells

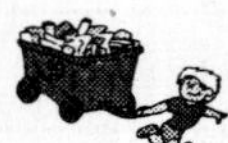

Natural Energy Resources

Part of the environment

- Fossil fuels
- Nuclear energy
- Hydroelectric power
- Solar
- Geo-thermal
- Wind
- Hydrogen

Other Types of Environments

Health environmental advocate promotes the following environments

1. Natural environment
2. Visual environment
3. Social-emotional environment

Chapter 14

Environmental Health

Chapter 15

Injury Prevention and Safety

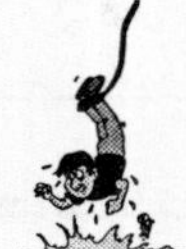

Unintentional Injuries – Accidental

- At home
  - Falls
  - Fires
  - Poisoning
  - Suffocation

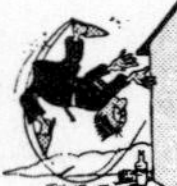

Unintentional Injuries – Accidental (cont'd)

- In the community
  - Drownings
  - Bicycle injuries
  - Scooter injuries

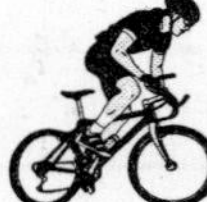

Unintentional Injuries – Accidental (cont'd)

- At the workplace
  - Use of machines and equipment
  - Driving
  - Homicide
  - Repetitive strain

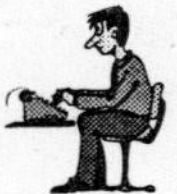

Occupational Safety & Health Act (OSHA) provides minimum safety standards

Natural Disasters

- Landslides
- Floods
- Earthquakes
- Tornadoes
- Hurricanes
- Wild fires
- Electrical storms
- Winter storms

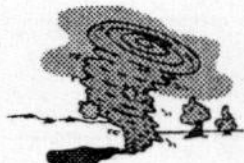

Motor Vehicle Safety

- Obtain proper authorization to drive
- Be a defensive driver
- Avoid high risk driving
- Avoid alcohol and driving

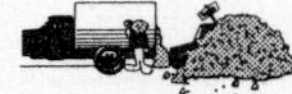

Motor Vehicle Safety (cont'd)

- Avoid violating traffic laws
- Wear a seatbelt
- Recognize "road rage"

Recognize Risks for Violence

- Bullying
- Fighting
- Assault
- Homicide
- Suicide
- Sexual harassment
- Rape
- Child abuse

Developing a Moral Code

- Set of rules that guide behavior
- 3 stages
  - *Stage 1: childhood* - develop a conscience
  - *Stage 2: adolescence* - develop conformity (right vs. wrong)
  - *Stage 3: adult* - commit to a set of principles (respect)

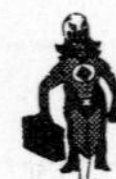

Self Protection Concepts

- Random violence
- Self-protection strategies
- Stalking
- Gangs
- Use of weapons

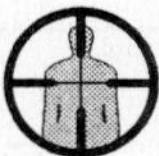

First Aid Procedures and Guidelines

- First aid kits
- Emergency numbers
- "Good Samaritan laws"
- Universal precautions
- How to check victim

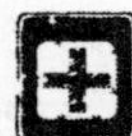

First Aid Procedures and Guidelines (cont'd)

- Choking emergencies
- Rescue breathing techniques
- CPR guidelines (heart attack/stroke)
- Stopping bleeding and other wounds
- Treating shock

First Aid
Procedures and Guidelines (cont'd)

- Poisoning procedures
- Animal/insect bites
- Burns
- Broken bones and joint injuries
- Environmental exposure

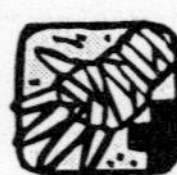

Chapter 15

Injury Prevention and Safety

Chapter 16

Using the Totally Awesome Teaching Strategies®

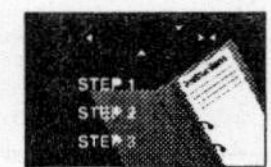

Teaching Strategies

- Techniques
- Help students understand concept
- Develop a specific skill

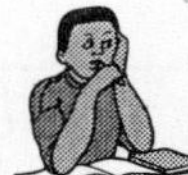

Totally Awesome Teaching Strategies

- Clever title
- Content area
- Specific grade level
- Infusion of other subject
- Health literacy

Totally Awesome Teaching Strategies (cont'd)

- Health standards
- Performance indicators
- Life goals
- Materials

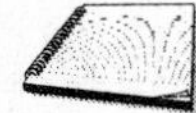

Totally Awesome Teaching Strategies (cont'd)

- Motivation
- Evaluation
- Multi-cultural infusion
- Inclusion

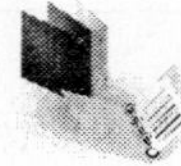

Grade Level: Kindergarten

Topic areas that should address the Totally Awesome Teaching Strategies

- Mental/emotional health
- Family/social health
- Growth & development
- Nutrition
- Personal health/ physical activity
- Alcohol, tobacco, and other drugs
- Communicable/ chronic diseases
- Consumer/ community health
- Environmental health
- Injury prevention and safety

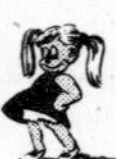

Grade Level: One

Topic areas that should address the Totally Awesome Teaching Strategies

- Mental/emotional health
- Family/social health
- Growth & development
- Nutrition
- Personal health/ physical activity
- Alcohol, tobacco, and other drugs
- Communicable/ chronic diseases
- Consumer/ community health
- Environmental health
- Injury prevention and safety

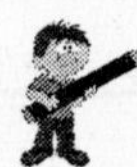

Grade Level: Two

Topic areas that should address the Totally Awesome Teaching Strategies

- Mental/emotional health
- Family/social health
- Growth & development
- Nutrition
- Personal health/ physical activity
- Alcohol, tobacco, and other drugs
- Communicable/ chronic diseases
- Consumer/ community health
- Environmental health
- Injury prevention and safety

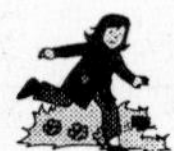

Grade Level: Three

Topic areas that should address the Totally Awesome Teaching Strategies

- Mental/emotional health
- Family/social health
- Growth & development
- Nutrition
- Personal health/ physical activity
- Alcohol, tobacco, and other drugs
- Communicable/ chronic diseases
- Consumer/ community health
- Environmental health
- Injury prevention and safety

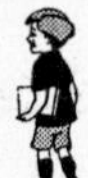

Grade Level: Four

Topic areas that should address the Totally Awesome Teaching Strategies

- Mental/emotional health
- Family/social health
- Growth & development
- Nutrition
- Personal health/ physical activity
- Alcohol, tobacco, and other drugs
- Communicable/ chronic diseases
- Consumer/ community health
- Environmental health
- Injury prevention and safety

Grade Level: Five

Topic areas that should address the Totally Awesome Teaching Strategies

- Mental/emotional health
- Family/social health
- Growth & development
- Nutrition
- Personal health/ physical activity
- Alcohol, tobacco, and other drugs
- Communicable/ chronic diseases
- Consumer/ community health
- Environmental health
- Injury prevention and safety

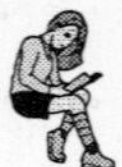

Grade Level: Six

Topic areas that should address the Totally Awesome Teaching Strategies

- Mental/emotional health
- Family/social health
- Growth & development
- Nutrition
- Personal health/ physical activity
- Alcohol, tobacco, and other drugs
- Communicable/ chronic diseases
- Consumer/ community health
- Environmental health
- Injury prevention and safety

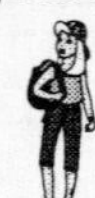

Grade Level: Seven

Topic areas that should address the Totally Awesome Teaching Strategies

- Mental/emotional health
- Family/social health
- Growth & development
- Nutrition
- Personal health/ physical activity
- Alcohol, tobacco, and other drugs
- Communicable/ chronic diseases
- Consumer/ community health
- Environmental health
- Injury prevention and safety

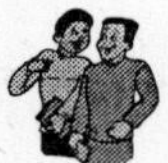

Grade Level: Eight

Topic areas that should address the Totally Awesome Teaching Strategies

- Mental/emotional health
- Family/social health
- Growth & development
- Nutrition
- Personal health/ physical activity
- Alcohol, tobacco, and other drugs
- Communicable/ chronic diseases
- Consumer/ community health
- Environmental health
- Injury prevention and safety

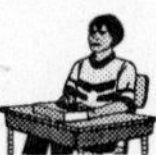

Grade Levels: Nine – Twelve

Topic areas that should address the Totally Awesome Teaching Strategies

- Mental/emotional health
- Family/social health
- Growth & development
- Nutrition
- Personal health/ physical activity
- Alcohol, tobacco, and other drugs
- Communicable/ chronic diseases
- Consumer/ community health
- Environmental health
- Injury prevention and safety

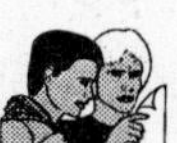

Chapter 16

Using the Totally Awesome Teaching Strategies®

Chapter 17

The Health Resource Guide

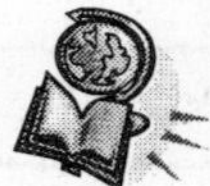

The Health Resource Guide

- Listing of organizations and agencies
- Phone numbers
- Websites
- Provides resources for assisting with school health education

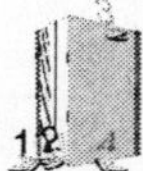

Resource Areas

1. Mental and emotional health
2. Family and social health
3. Growth and development
4. Nutrition

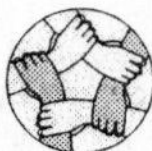

Resource Areas (cont'd)

5. Personal health and physical activity
6. Alcohol, tobacco and other drugs
7. Communicable and chronic health
8. Environmental health

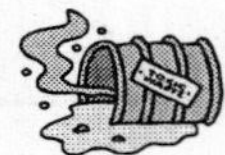

Resource Areas (cont'd)

9. Injury prevention and safety
10. Consumer and community health
11. Professional health organizations
12. Related national organizations

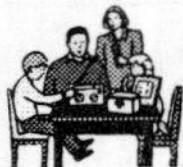

Organizations and Associations

- Should also provide the following:
  - *Free, inexpensive materials (i.e., pamphlets, kits, videos)*
  - *Services (i.e., speakers, support groups, other programs)*
  - *Hotlines (24 hour access)*
  - *Careers and job opportunities*

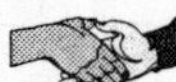

Chapter 17

The Health Resource Guide

Chapter 18

Using the Meeks Heit K-12 Health Education Curriculum Guide

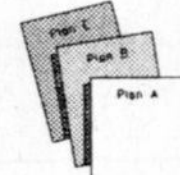

Comprehensive School Health Education Curriculum

- Sequential K-12 plan
- Promotes health literacy
- Components necessary for successful health program

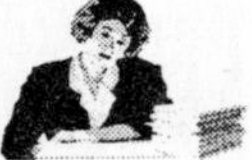

Meeks Heit K-12 Health Education Curriculum Guide

- Goals and philosophy
- National Health Education Standard (NHES)
  - *One: Comprehend health information*
  - *Two: Access valid health information, products, and services*
  - *Three: Practice healthful behaviors*
  - *Four: Analyze influences on health*

Meeks Heit K-12 Health Education Curriculum Guide (cont'd)

- National Health Education Standard (NHES)
  - *Five: Use communication, resistance, and skills conflict resolution*
  - *Six: Set health goals and make responsible decisions*
  - *Seven: Be a health advocate*

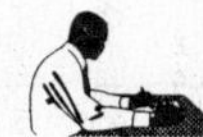

Meeks Heit K-12 Health Education Curriculum Guide (cont'd)

- National Health Education Standard (NHES)
  - *1-7: Demonstrate good character*
  - *Abstinence education*
  - *Totally awesome teaching strategies*
  - *Children's literature*

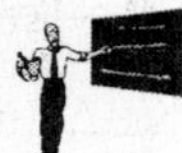

Meeks Heit K-12 Health Education Curriculum Guide (cont'd)

- National Health Education Standard (NHES)
  - *Curriculum infusion*
  - *Health literacy*
  - *Inclusion of students with special needs*
  - *Service learning*

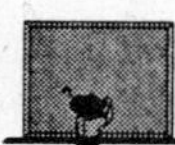

Meeks Heit K-12 Health Education Curriculum Guide (cont'd)

- National Health Education Standard (NHES)
  - *Multi-cultural infusion*
  - *Family involvement*
  - *Evaluation*
  - *The Meeks Heit K-12 scope and sequence chart*

Chapter 18

Using the Meeks Heit K-12 Health Education Curriculum Guide